Growing You

**KEEPSAKE PREGNANCY JOURNAL AND
MEMORY BOOK FOR MOM AND BABY**

Korie Herold

paige tate & CO.

Copyright © Korie Herold
Published in 2020 by Blue Star Press
Paige Tate & Co. is an imprint of Blue Star Press
PO Box 8835, Bend, OR 97708
contact@paigetate.com | www.paigetate.com

Illustrations and Design by Korie Herold

ISBN: 9781944515973
Printed in China
10 9 8 7 6 5 4 3

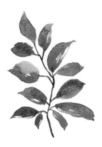

To the brave women who journey into motherhood, may your stories live on beyond this season of beautiful growth.

Each page of this book was delicately crafted, illustrated, and painted by hand by a single artist located in Kingwood, TX. Learn more about the artist behind this journal at the end of the book.

ABOUT THIS JOURNAL

This is your pregnancy story, and it's important to me that you get to tell it exactly as it happened, since no journey is exactly the same. I created this journal as a place to document your innermost thoughts and experiences of bringing new life into the world, no matter how your story unfolds. This journal is meant to be customized as if it was made just for you.

Growing You is a place to celebrate and document this most special time in your life as a mother, reflecting on the growth, anticipation, and memories that you want to hold on to. The spiral binding allows you to customize this journal specifically to your story; simply remove any pages you may wish to not include, or that do not apply to you. For example, if you don't make the full term of pregnancy, simply remove the pages after the month you made it to, and the pages will flow straight into your birth plan and birth story. If you need to remove pages, I recommend that you do so with the careful use of scissors, rather than tearing out pages by hand.

To get the most out of your journal, there is a pocket in the back to hold cherished mementos from this special season of motherhood: sonograms, cards for baby, maternity photographs, and so on. Think about what a beautiful piece of history you are creating for your child with this journal, to one day pass along to them to learn about their first days.

For quality and consistency, I recommend that you use a black archival ink pen instead of a ballpoint pen. I use Micron pens.

I would love to see you using Growing You during your pregnancy! Use the hashtag #GrowingYouJournal to connect on social media.

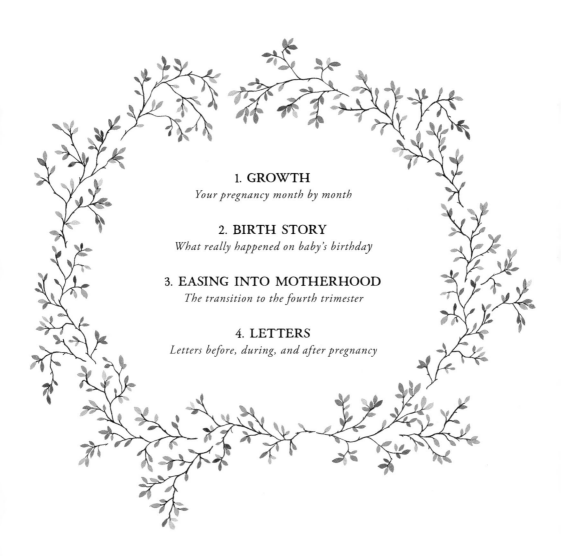

TABLE OF CONTENTS

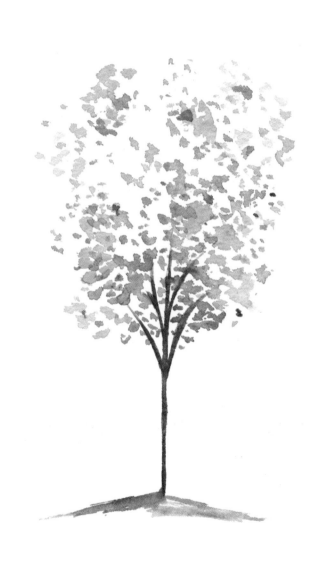

Growth

Use this section of *Growing You* to document your monthly growth during pregnancy. Also included is a set of pages for family and friends to guess the gender of your baby before their arrival.

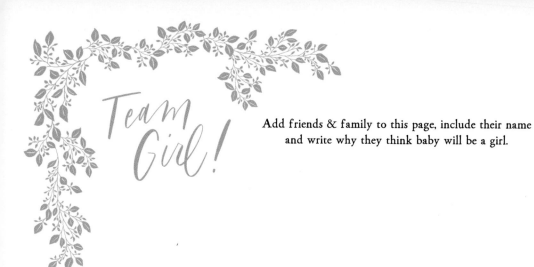

Team Girl!

Add friends & family to this page, include their name and write why they think baby will be a girl.

Add friends & family to this page, include their name
and write why they think baby will be a boy.

Team Boy!

Current Guidelines for a Healthy Pregnancy

For example : Avoid lunch meat and raw sushi, "back is best," etc.

- Get a lot of rest
- eat a nutritious diet (mommy always craves fruit)
- no sushi or lunch meat
- wear mask and wash hands (COVID-19)
- Don't pick up a new exercise routine
- Take good care of your gums (mine have been very sensitive)

Prenatal Appointments

Date : **1/6/2021**
- Dr. confirmed our pregnancy
- ordered first ultrasound
- original due date: sept. 2nd (grandma's birthday!)

Date :

Date : **1/13/2021**
- first ultrasound
- changed due date to August 17th (another Leo in the family)

Date :

Date : **2/3/2021**
- answered our questions
- did some blood work (mom is O+ and Dad is A+)
- mom and baby are healthy!

Date :

Date :

Date :

Suggested information to include : doctor/midwife/doula, dilation, measurements, weight, week, progress, etc.

Prenatal Appointments

Date : _____

Date : _____

Date : _____

Date : _____

Date : _____

Date : _____

Date : _____

Date : _____

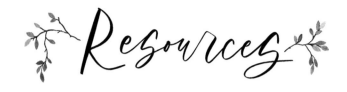

Resources

Websites, books, groups, apps, and other resources I found helpful during pregnancy.

- What to Expect When You're Expecting
  ↑ my bible ↑
- Baby center App
- What to expect App
- Kinder (like Tinder for baby names, swipe left and right)

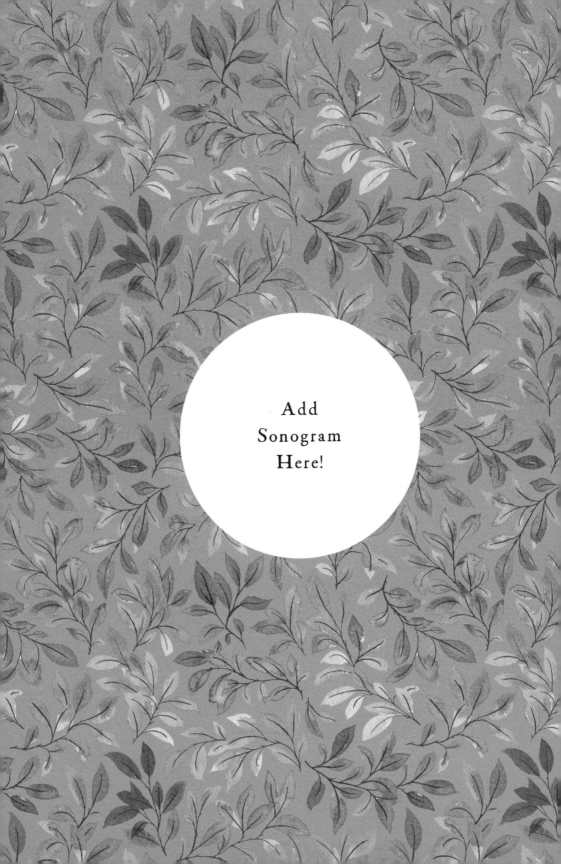

Add
Sonogram
Here!

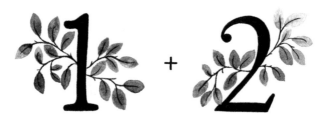

months : the early days

Three words to describe pregnancy : ....
....

I'm nervous about : ....
....
....

I'm excited about : ....
....
....

Things I'm craving lately : ....
....
....

My nickname for you : ....
....

You are now the size of : ....
....

Ways my body has changed : _____

_____

_____

_____

How I would describe my sleep : _____

_____

_____

_____

Reflecting on this time of being pregnant with you : _____

_____

_____

_____

How I feel : _____

_____

_____

_____

Pregnancy dreams : _____

_____

_____

_____

I was here when I first found out I was pregnant with you : _____

_____

I had a feeling I was pregnant because : _____

_____

The first person besides me to know about you was : _____

This is how I told that person : _____

_____

_____

_____

This is how long we kept the pregnancy a secret : _____

_____

_____

_____

This is what the first doctor appointment/ultrasound was like : _____

_____

_____

_____

_____

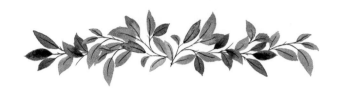

Thoughts, reflections, or stories from this past month : ....

....

....

....

....

....

....

....

....

....

....

....

....

....

....

....

....

....

....

....

....

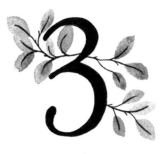

months

Three words to describe pregnancy : _____

_____

I'm nervous about : _____

_____

_____

I'm excited about : _____

_____

_____

Things I'm craving lately : _____

_____

_____

My nickname for you : _____

_____

You are now the size of : _____

_____

Ways my body has changed : _____

_____

_____

_____

How I would describe my sleep : _____

_____

_____

_____

_____

Reflecting on this time of being pregnant with you : _____

_____

_____

_____

_____

How I feel : _____

_____

_____

_____

Pregnancy dreams : _____

_____

_____

_____

Is the pregnancy still a secret? Who knows right now? How was the news shared?

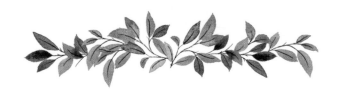

Thoughts, reflections, or stories from this past month : _____

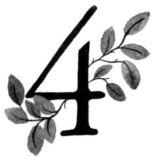

months

Three words to describe pregnancy : ....
....

I'm nervous about : ....
....
....

I'm excited about : ....
....
....

Things I'm craving lately : ....
....
....

My nickname for you : ....
....

You are now the size of : ....
....

Ways my body has changed : _____

_____

_____

_____

_____

How I would describe my sleep : _____

_____

_____

_____

_____

Reflecting on this time of being pregnant with you : _____

_____

_____

_____

_____

How I feel : _____

_____

_____

_____

_____

Pregnancy dreams : _____

_____

_____

_____

_____

Have I started showing?

Plans and feelings on finding out (or waiting to know) the gender :

What I think about most in this stage of my pregnancy :

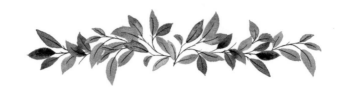

Thoughts, reflections, or stories from this past month : _____

_____

_____

_____

_____

_____

_____

_____

_____

_____

_____

_____

_____

_____

_____

_____

_____

_____

_____

_____

_____

_____

months

Three words to describe pregnancy : _____

_____

I'm nervous about : _____

_____

_____

I'm excited about : _____

_____

_____

Things I'm craving lately : _____

_____

_____

My nickname for you : _____

_____

You are now the size of : _____

_____

Ways my body has changed : _____

_____

_____

_____

How I would describe my sleep : _____

_____

_____

_____

Reflecting on this time of being pregnant with you : _____

_____

_____

_____

How I feel : _____

_____

_____

_____

Pregnancy dreams : _____

_____

_____

_____

20-week ultrasound appointment :

I found out your gender. Here was my reaction :

I did not find out your gender, but my hunch is that you are :

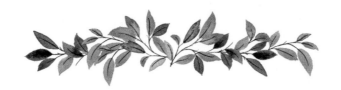

Thoughts, reflections, or stories from this past month : _____

months

Three words to describe pregnancy : ....

....

I'm nervous about : ....

....

....

I'm excited about : ....

....

....

Things I'm craving lately : ....

....

....

My nickname for you : ....

....

You are now the size of : ....

....

Ways my body has changed : _____

_____

_____

_____

How I would describe my sleep : _____

_____

_____

_____

Reflecting on this time of being pregnant with you : _____

_____

_____

_____

How I feel : _____

_____

_____

_____

Pregnancy dreams : _____

_____

_____

_____

Names that are in the running :

Characteristics I hope you get from me :

Traits I hope to instill in you :

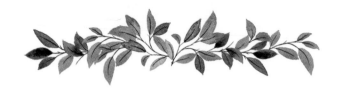

Thoughts, reflections, or stories from this past month : ....
....

....

....

....

....

....

....

....

....

....

....

....

....

....

....

....

....

....

....

....

....

....

....

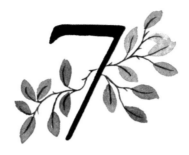

months

Three words to describe pregnancy : ....

....

I'm nervous about : ....

....

....

I'm excited about : ....

....

....

Things I'm craving lately : ....

....

....

My nickname for you : ....

....

You are now the size of : ....

....

Ways my body has changed : _____

_____

_____

_____

_____

How I would describe my sleep : _____

_____

_____

_____

Reflecting on this time of being pregnant with you : _____

_____

_____

_____

How I feel : _____

_____

_____

_____

Pregnancy dreams : _____

_____

_____

_____

Funny comments people have made to me about pregnancy : ....

Who I think you'll most look like when you are born : ....

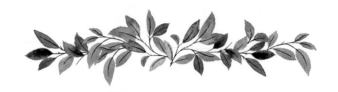

Thoughts, reflections, or stories from this past month : ....

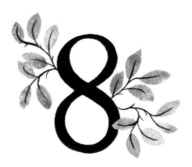

months

Three words to describe pregnancy : ....

....

I'm nervous about : ....

....

....

I'm excited about : ....

....

....

Things I'm craving lately : ....

....

....

My nickname for you : ....

....

You are now the size of : ....

....

Ways my body has changed : _____

_____

_____

_____

_____

How I would describe my sleep : _____

_____

_____

_____

_____

Reflecting on this time of being pregnant with you : _____

_____

_____

_____

_____

How I feel : _____

_____

_____

_____

_____

Pregnancy dreams : _____

_____

_____

_____

Thoughts on baby shower(s) :

My favorite gift I received for you is :

Adventures you have been on with me :

Parenting or birthing classes I took :

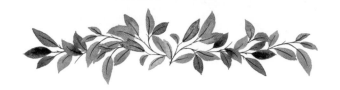

Thoughts, reflections, or stories from this past month : ....

months

Three words to describe pregnancy : _____
_____

I'm nervous about : _____
_____
_____

I'm excited about : _____
_____
_____

Things I'm craving lately : _____
_____
_____

My nickname for you : _____
_____

You are now the size of : _____
_____

Ways my body has changed : _____

_____

_____

_____

_____

How I would describe my sleep : _____

_____

_____

_____

_____

Reflecting on this time of being pregnant with you : _____

_____

_____

_____

_____

How I feel : _____

_____

_____

_____

_____

Pregnancy dreams : _____

_____

_____

_____

How I would describe your nursery : ....

....

....

....

....

....

Special things I made just for you : ....

....

....

....

....

....

Other ways I prepared for your arrival : ....

....

....

....

....

....

....

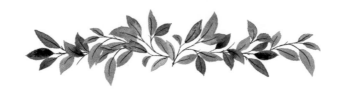

Thoughts, reflections, or stories from this past month :

Birth plan

Birth plan

Birth Story

Use this section of *Growing You* to document the story of
your baby's birth, including how it went, how you felt, who
was there with you, and other special memories.

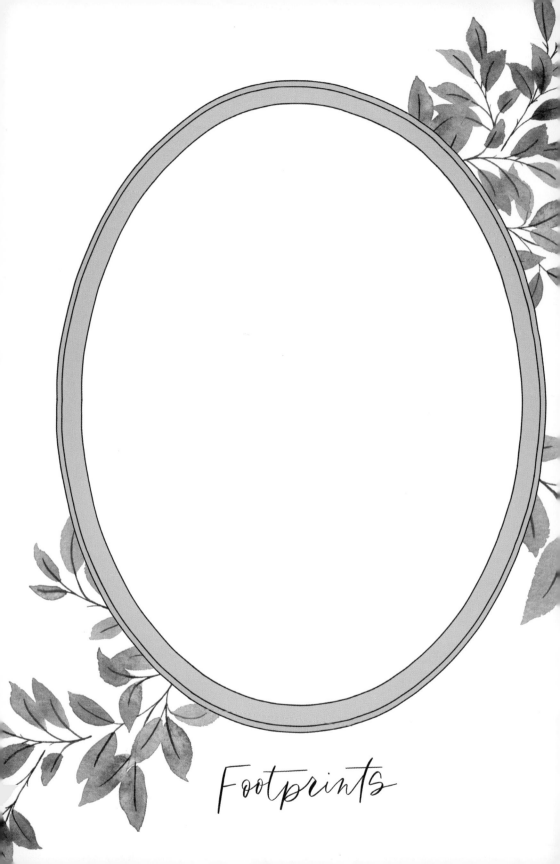

Footprints

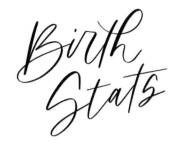

Birth Stats

Date : _____

Time : _____

Doctor/Midwife/Doula : _____

_____

Who was present awaiting your arrival? _____

_____

Place/City : _____

_____

Height : _____

Weight : _____

Hair : _____

Eyes : _____

Weather outside : _____

_____

_____

First words upon meeting you : _____

_____

_____

I was here when I knew you were coming : _____

_____

_____

_____

_____

These people were in the room when you were born : _____

_____

_____

_____

_____

Labor lasted this long : _____

_____

_____

_____

How I'd describe my labor with you : _____

_____

_____

_____

_____

_____

_____

_____

I immediately fell in love with this feature of yours :

These people came to visit us after your birth :

Your name, and how we decided on it for you :

How I felt when I first laid eyes on you :

Add Photo Here!

Your first outfit and why I picked it : _____

_____

_____

_____

_____

_____

Birth Story

Birth Story

Birth Story

Birth Story

Birth Story

Birth Story

Easing Into Motherhood

Use this section of *Growing You* to document your feelings
and experiences during your first days and weeks of motherhood.

My first real night with you, without any help from the hospital/birthing center, or doula, was like this :

How I'd describe our sleep lately :

You sleep here these days :

My healing process from giving birth :

These are the moments with you that bring me bliss : _____

_____

_____

_____

_____

_____

_____

_____

This still makes me nervous : _____

_____

_____

_____

_____

_____

_____

_____

_____

_____

_____

Early difficulties I'm trying to figure out :

Help from others I received after your birth :

Additional thoughts about easing into motherhood :

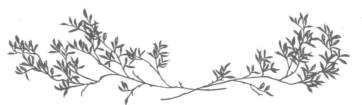

Letters

This section of *Growing You* is open-ended and completely up to you as to how you want to use it. The blue banner ribbon on the crest of each journal page is intended to house the date you are writing. Consider writing letters to yourself, writing letters to baby, or using this section as a personal prayer journal. To get you started, here are a few ideas for how you might want to use these pages :

- A letter to yourself about pregnancy

- A letter to yourself about giving birth

- A letter to yourself about becoming a mom

- A letter to yourself about healing

- A letter about a lesson that was hard to learn

- A letter about how you changed after baby's arrival

- A letter of gratefulness

- A letter of hopes for baby's future

- A letter for high school graduation

- A letter for leaving the nest

- A letter to baby's future spouse

- A letter of advice

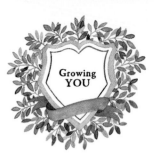

Growing
YOU

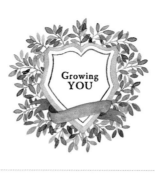

Growing
YOU

Growing
YOU

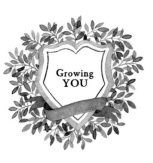

Growing
YOU

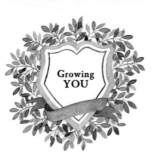

Growing
YOU

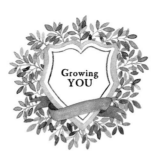

Growing
YOU

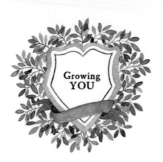

Growing
YOU

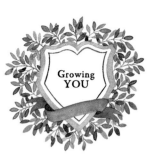

Growing
YOU

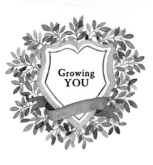

Growing
YOU

Growing
YOU

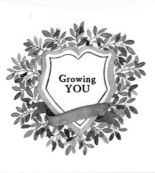

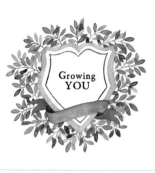

Growing
YOU

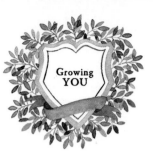

Growing
YOU

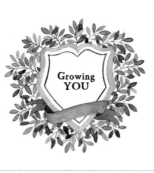

Growing
YOU

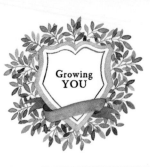

Growing
YOU

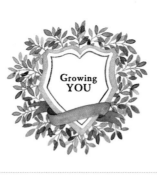

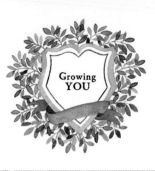

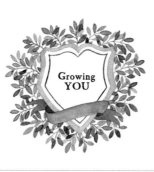

Growing
YOU

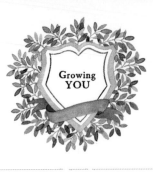

Growing
YOU

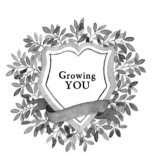

Growing
YOU

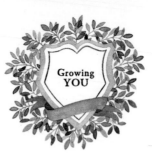

Growing
YOU

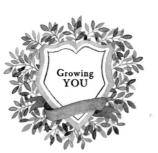

Growing
YOU

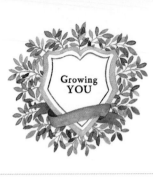

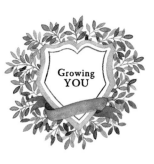

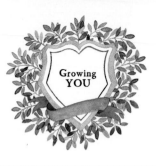

Hi! I'm Korie

Wow, what a privilege it is for me to get to pour my heart into a journal that allows women to tell such a personal story within its pages. I'm so grateful you picked up this journal and deemed it worthy to hold your most precious thoughts and experiences. I pray this becomes a treasured part of your pregnancy as you grow physically and mentally, preparing for the chapters that lie ahead. Should your story unfold differently than you hoped for, let this journal be a safe space for you to process that experience as well.

I'd love the opportunity to connect with you in another way, and introduce you to my work. I've created a free download of additional letter writing pages and printable artwork that can be found at:

www.korieherold.com/free

SPECIAL THANKS

My husband—I'm looking at you, Joel. Your constant support and encouragement to keep on creating is what keeps me going. You fuel my fire and I'm so grateful for you. Thank you for creating a safe space for me to chase my dreams, one after the next.

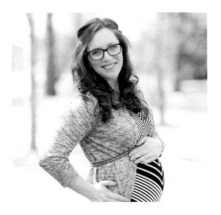

Paige Tate & Co.—Thank you for consistently encouraging me to create books I want to see more of in the world. You know this wouldn't be possible without you. I am so grateful you answered my email all those years ago and said "yes" to this journey with me. Thank you for allowing my voice and vision to shine through, and more importantly, thank you for your friendship along the way. Y'all are the best kind of people.

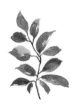

Growing You

KEEPSAKE PREGNANCY JOURNAL AND
MEMORY BOOK FOR MOM AND BABY

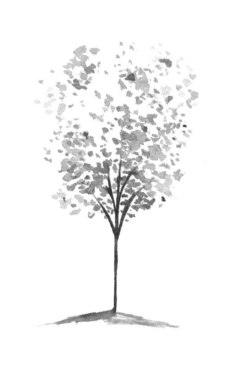

Inside This Pocket